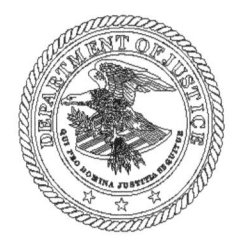

Department of Justice

I0503292

STATEMENT OF

JOSEPH T. RANNAZZISI
DEPUTY ASSISTANT ADMINISTRATOR
OFFICE OF DIVERSION CONTROL
DRUG ENFORCEMENT ADMINISTRATION

BEFORE THE

CAUCUS ON INTERNATIONAL NARCOTICS CONTROL
UNITED STATES SENATE

FOR A HEARING ENTITLED

"DANGEROUS SYNTHETIC DRUGS"

PRESENTED ON

SEPTEMBER 25, 2013

Statement of Joseph T. Rannazzisi
Deputy Assistant Administrator, Office of Diversion Control
Drug Enforcement Administration
United States Department of Justice

Before the Senate Caucus on International Narcotics Control
For a Hearing Entitled "Dangerous Synthetic Drugs"
September 25, 2013

Chairman Feinstein, Co-Chairman Grassley, and distinguished members of the Caucus on International Narcotics Control, on behalf of Administrator Leonhart and the Drug Enforcement Administration (DEA), I appreciate your invitation to testify today regarding DEA's efforts to combat the emerging challenges presented by synthetic cannabinoids and stimulants.

Designer Drugs – Historical Perspective

"Throughout the drug discovery process, pharmaceutical companies, academic institutions, research institutions, and other organizations publish their studies in scientific journals, books and patents. This information exchange, which is essential to the legitimate scientific enterprise, can be, and is, used by clandestine chemists who duplicate the technical sophistication used by the research community to manufacture and market a seemingly endless variety of analogs of so-called designer drugs."[1]

The term "designer drug" is a colloquial term that references substances with properties and effects similar to those of stimulant, depressant, hallucinogenic or narcotic drugs but that are chemically modified to evade control as an illicit drug. Although news reports tend to portray the appearance of these substances as a new trend, designer drugs have been in the illicit marketplace for decades. The distinction of today's designer drugs is the substantial volume and endless variety of designer drugs easily available to the public and the organized, extensive distribution networks utilized by designer drug traffickers.

Since the 1970s, domestic clandestine chemists have attempted to manipulate the molecular structures of controlled substances to create synthetic drugs that would have the same pharmacologic properties of a controlled drug, but not expose the chemist or distributor to criminal violations under the Federal Controlled Substances Act (CSA) or similar state statutes. Since these drugs are created in a clandestine laboratory, no manufacturing standards or safety and efficacy studies, such as those required by the Food and Drug Administration (FDA) with

---

[1] F. Ivy Carroll, Anita H. Lewin, S. Wayne Mascarella, Herbert H. Seltzman, and P. Anantha Reddy. Designer drugs: a medicinal chemistry perspective. *Annals of the New York Academy of Sciences* 2012, 1248, 18-38.

respect to pharmaceutical drugs, ensure the safety of the products ingested. Designer drugs were distinguished from traditional illicit drugs of abuse due to the lack of history and appreciation for the short and long-term health effects of use. Historically, the introduction of "designer drugs" into the marketplace was generally similar to that of illicit controlled substances: covert meetings and sales on street corners, back alleys, and in dark clubs. During this time period, the infusion of these drugs into the illicit marketplace wreaked havoc in certain areas of the country.

In the 1970s and 1980s, clandestine chemists introduced synthetic alternatives to the Schedule II drug fentanyl into the illicit marketplace. These drugs were distributed to heroin abusers who were unaware that the drug they were purchasing was 100 to 500 times more potent than morphine. Drug abusers were the unknowing test subjects used to determine the viability of the substances as a replacement for controlled narcotics. This uncontrolled experimentation resulted in overdose deaths in concentrated areas of the country with law enforcement authorities scrambling to identify the drug and locate the clandestine laboratories and chemists that produced the substances. In some instances, it wasn't the strength of the drug, but its toxic contaminants that ultimately harmed the users. For example, a domestic chemist was attempting to manufacture MPPP, a synthetic alternative to the Schedule II drug meperidine (Demerol®). During the manufacturing process, the chemist manufactured MPPP that was contaminated with MPTP, a neurotoxin that caused end stage Parkinson's symptoms (involuntary motor movement) in the user. Again, the clandestine chemist was using illicit drug users as subjects for his own personal laboratory experiment, with tragic results. At the time, these synthesized drugs were not controlled substances under the CSA and therefore there was little, if any, criminal exposure and little incentive to stop manufacturing and producing the drugs. The possibility of synthesizing a non-controlled substance that could produce millions of dollars in income was too enticing to stop experimenting on a readily-available number of test subjects.

Congress responded in 1986 by passing the Controlled Substance Analogue Enforcement Act (Analogue Act), which provides: "[a] controlled substance analogue shall, to the extent intended for human consumption, be treated . . . as a controlled substance in schedule I." 21 U.S.C. § 813. A "controlled substance analogue" means a substance:

> (i) the chemical structure of which is substantially similar to the chemical structure of a controlled substance in schedule I or II;

> (ii) which has a stimulant, depressant, or hallucinogenic effect on the central nervous system that is substantially similar to or greater than the stimulant, depressant, or hallucinogenic effect on the central nervous system of a controlled substance in schedule I or II; or

> (iii) with respect to a particular person, which such person represents or intends to have a stimulant, depressant, or hallucinogenic effect on the central nervous

system that is substantially similar to or greater than the stimulant, depressant, or hallucinogenic effect on the central nervous system of a controlled substance in schedule I or II.[2]

The Analogue Act provided law enforcement authorities with the authority to investigate and prosecute clandestine chemists who had been manufacturing and distributing dangerous drugs with impunity due to a loophole in the CSA. Historically, designer drugs were produced by a small number of sophisticated chemists in domestic clandestine laboratories located throughout the United States. Although it took time and resources to identify and locate the chemist and lab, the Analogue Act allowed law enforcement authorities to seize the drugs, chemicals and glassware/equipment, arrest and prosecute the chemist/violator, thus dismantling the manufacturing and distribution operation. The Analogue Act did not control designer drugs per se, but rather allowed certain substances to be treated as Schedule I controlled substances to the extent intended for human consumption. Criminal liability depends upon a finding, in each particular prosecution, that the substance is a "controlled substance analogue" and that the substance was intended for human consumption. This requires extensive use of expert witnesses to prove substantial structural similarity and similar pharmacologic effect. The Analogue Act answered the designer drug problem at that particular time in history--it provided law enforcement with the ability to stop small-scale, domestic clandestine chemists and their clandestine laboratories.

After the Analogue Act, law enforcement agencies continued to encounter synthetic drugs in the illicit market. In addition to non-controlled substances that could be treated as analogues of opioids, law enforcement agencies also encountered other non-controlled substances such as benzylpiperazine (BZP) and trifloromethylphenylpiperazine (TFMPP) that were sold in combination in order to mimic the effects of MDMA (ecstasy), which was controlled under Schedule I of the CSA in 1985. Other non-controlled substances included those sold as amphetamine substitutes, such as the hallucinogen 5-MeO-AMT, a substance that is widely regarded as an analogue of the Schedule I controlled substance AMT, from the tryptamine class of compounds, and methcathinone, which is widely regarded as an analogue of cathinone. Eventually, law enforcement authorities began to see a shift in which chemists began manufacturing MDMA, BZP and TFMPP in foreign clandestine laboratories and then smuggling the substances into the United States for distribution.

The Current Situation Concerning Designer Drugs

As discussed, traditional designer drugs such as opioids (e.g., 3-methyl fentanyl, alpha-methyl fentanyl) and stimulants (e.g., amphetamine, methamphetamine, methcathinone) were historically manufactured in clandestine laboratories in the United States. The new generation of

---

[2] 21 U.S.C. § 802(32).

designer drugs, such as synthetic cannabinoids (often marketed under the guise of herbal incense or potpourri), stimulants (e.g., cathinones often marketed under the guise of "bath salts") and hallucinogens (e.g., tryptamines, piperazines), are not predominantly synthesized in domestic clandestine laboratories. Instead, the vast majority of this new generation of designer drugs are developed and manufactured in foreign clandestine laboratories and then smuggled into the United States in bulk form or as finished product. The shift to large-scale foreign manufacture limits the deterrent effect of the Analogue Act as well as the ability of law enforcement authorities to proactively identify and prevent potential designer drug threats. Instead, law enforcement authorities must wait for the next new designer drug to be identified after it is smuggled into the United States and sold in retail environments with inconspicuous labeling. As a result, abusers and unsuspecting youth have been exposed to the dangerous substances and, in many instances, have even suffered adverse health consequences, including death.

The National Forensic Laboratory Information System (NFLIS) is a national repository for drug identification results from analyses conducted by forensic laboratories across the United States. NFLIS shows that synthetic cannabinoids, stimulants and hallucinogens have taken over the designer drug market and abusers are seeking these substances as alternatives to traditionally illicit drugs of abuse. In 2009, NFLIS contained 15 synthetic cannabinoid reports related to two different substances and 34 synthetic cathinone reports representing four different substances. By 2011, the number of reports for synthetic cannabinoids was greater than the number of reports for synthetic cathinones, tryptamines, piperazines and 2C-phenethylamines combined. By 2012, the number of synthetic cannabinoid exhibit reports exceeded 41,200 and related to 56 different cannabinoids, far greater than the other classes of designer drugs. Synthetic cathinones were not as popular as synthetic cannabinoids, with 14,100 reports representing 31 different cathinones. Of particular concern, the synthetic cannabinoid AM-2201 ranked 8th overall out of the top 10 drugs reported to NFLIS with over 14,200 reports—approximately the same number of reports as all synthetic cathinones in that year.

NFLIS also shows that other designer drugs are gaining popularity. From 2007 to 2009, NFLIS reported an increase in reports of piperazines and tryptamines sent to local, state, and Federal analytical laboratories throughout the country. The piperazine and tryptamine classes of drugs have psychoactive properties and are generally sold as substitutes for ecstasy (MDMA) or other hallucinogens.

The designer drug problem is growing globally as well. In 2012, the United Nations Office on Drugs and Crime (UNODC) conducted the first comprehensive survey of a number of U.N. member states looking at the synthetic drug (or "New Psychoactive Substance (NPS)" as it is referred to by the international community) problem; some 80 countries and territories, from all regions of the world, provided data on the emergence of NPS. Over 85% of the nations surveyed (70 out of 80) indicated that NPS had appeared on their drug market.

Designer Drugs of Concern

Currently, synthetic cannabinoids, synthetic stimulants (including phenethylamines such as synthetic cathinones), piperazines, and tryptamines are designer drugs that are manufactured and distributed on a large scale, and are marketed in a manner to avoid liability under the CSA. The manufacturers and retailers who make and sell these products do not disclose all of the product ingredients, including the active and potentially harmful ingredient(s). Designer drugs today are often marketed in a manner intended to mask their intended purpose and are, consequently, often labeled as "not for human consumption," or "for novelty use only." These statements are intended to frustrate the application of the Analogue Act, which states that controlled substance analogues shall, *"to the extent intended for human consumption,"* be treated as a controlled substance in Schedule I. 21 U.S.C. § 813 (emphasis added).

Historically, the introduction of designer drugs into the marketplace was generally similar to that of illicit controlled substances: covert meetings and sales on street corners, back alleys, and in dark clubs. In many instances, the ingestion of these drugs led to tragedy. Today however, the marketing of designer drugs has ushered in a new era of drug distribution. No longer are these substances sold in a covert manner to avoid detection by law enforcement authorities. Instead, the substances are sold openly on the shelves at gas stations, convenience stores, head shops, and via the Internet from both domestic and international sources. At retail establishments, they are sold in plain view with disclaimers such as "not for human consumption," in products masquerading as incense, potpourri, bath salts, plant food, glass/window and jewelry cleaner, badger repellant, and snail/slug repellant. Substances as dangerous as their controlled substance equivalents are marketed as harmless sundry items in an attempt to shield the manufacturers, distributors and retail sellers from criminal prosecution. This type of marketing is nothing more than a means to make dangerous, psychoactive substances widely-available to the public.

Synthetic Cannabinoids (Herbal Incense Products)

Background and History

Synthetic cannabinoids are a large family of compounds that are functionally (biologically) similar to THC, the main active ingredient in marijuana. Synthetic cannabinoids, however, are not organic but are chemicals created in a laboratory. Two of the synthetic cannabinoids currently controlled (CP-47,497 and cannabicyclohexanol) were first synthesized in the early 1980's for research purposes in the investigation of the cannabinoid system. JWH-018, JWH-073, and JWH-200 (all controlled under the Synthetic Drug Abuse Prevention Act of 2012) were synthesized in the mid-1990s and studied to further advance the understanding of drug-receptor interactions regarding the cannabinoid system. Synthesized as research tools, no other known legitimate uses have been identified for these five synthetic cannabinoids.

According to forensic laboratory reports, the initial appearance of synthetic cannabinoids in herbal incense products in the United States occurred in November 2008 when U.S. Customs and Border Protection first encountered products using brand names such as "Spice." Prior to appearing on the U.S. market, synthetic cannabinoids were marketed in herbal incense products in several European countries. After experiencing numerous health-related incidents, some European countries banned these products/chemicals. According to U.S. Customs and Border Protection, a number of the synthetic cannabinoids appeared to originate from foreign sources.

Detailed chemical analyses by DEA and other agencies have found these synthetic cannabinoids laced on plant material in herbal incense products marketed to the general public. Product analyses have found variations in both the type of synthetic cannabinoid and the amount of the substance found on the plant material.

The vast majority of cannabinoids are manufactured in Asia by foreign chemists who are not bound by any manufacturing requirements or quality control standards. The bulk products are smuggled into the United States typically as misbranded imports. These chemicals are generally found in powder form or are dissolved in solvents, such as acetone, before being applied to the plant material comprising the "herbal incense" products. After local distributors apply the drug to the leafy material, they package it for retail distribution, again ignoring any control mechanisms to prevent contamination or to ensure a consistent, uniform concentration of drug in each package. According to Internet discussion boards and law enforcement encounters, spraying or mixing the synthetic cannabinoids on plant material provides a vehicle for the most common route of administration - smoking (using a pipe, a water pipe, or rolling the drug-spiked plant material in cigarette papers). They are sold under hundreds of different brand names, including "Spice," "K2," "Blaze," "Red X Dawn," "Paradise," "Demon," "Black Magic," "Spike," "Mr. Nice Guy," "Ninja," " Zohai," "Dream," "Genie," "Sence," "Smoke," "Skunk," "Serenity," "Yucatan," "Fire," and "Crazy Clown."

Law enforcement personnel have encountered dosage form and packaging operations in residential neighborhoods, garages, and warehouses. Throughout this process, there is no concern for preventing contamination of the product, consistent dosage, or the adverse health consequences that may occur from ingesting the drug. As proposed in scientific literature, the risk of adverse health effects is further increased by the fact that similar products vary in the composition and concentration of synthetic cannabinoids laced on the plant material. The user is unwittingly a guinea pig in an uncontrolled laboratory test and the consequences can be deadly.

The popularity of synthetic cannabinoids has significantly increased throughout the United States over the last five years because of their psychoactive properties as reported by law enforcement agencies, the medical community, and in scientific literature. The widespread use of these drugs may be due to their accessibility and availability, the perception that these substances are "legal" alternatives to illicit drugs, and that they provide a pharmacologic affect similar to that of illicit drugs when smoked. Even though synthetic cannabinoids are marketed as "herbal incense" products, there is no evidence that these synthetic cannabinoids add value to genuine incense products—there is no scent or odor associated with these substances.

The widespread retail sale of these products provides persons of all ages with direct access to synthetic cannabinoids and the corresponding THC-like effects of these products. Research articles propose that the packaging is professional and conspicuous and targets young people, possibly eager to use cannabis, but who are afraid of the legal consequences and/or association with illicit drugs. In fact, these drugs have become increasingly popular, particularly among teens and young adults because of the perceived legality of the substances. They are also popular among those individuals who are subject to urinalysis testing, such as those individuals who are under the supervision of a drug court and those on probation or parole.

Recent surveys confirm the widespread, continued use of synthetic cannabinoids (also known as "synthetic marijuana") by youth. In the annual survey *Monitoring the Future*, 11.3 percent of 12th graders reported past year synthetic cannabinoid use in 2012 in comparison to 11.4 percent of 12th graders in 2011.[3] For 2010, Drug Abuse Warning Network (DAWN) reported an estimated 11,406 emergency department (ED) visits involved a synthetic cannabinoid product.[4] From this same report, *Drug-Related Emergency Department Visits Involving Synthetic Cannabinoids*, three-fourths (75 percent or 8,557) of the 2010 estimated ED visits involved patients 12 to 29 years of age. The estimated 8,557 visits for patients aged 12 to 29 includes 3,780 estimated ED visits for patients aged 12 to 17, 33 percent of 11,406 total ED visits. In the majority (59 percent) of these ED visits for patients 12 to 29 years of age, synthetic cannabinoids were involved alone with no other substances. Synthetic cannabinoids appeared for the first time at reportable levels in the DAWN in 2010, when they were involved in 11,406 estimated ED visits (1.0 percent of all ED visits involving illicit drugs). In 2011, DAWN reported a total of 28,531 estimated ED visits, or 2.35 percent of all ED visits involving illicit drugs, involved synthetic cannabinoids.[5]

Adverse Effects

Self-reported abuse of synthetic cannabinoids appears extensively on Internet discussion boards, and abuse has been reported to public health officials and law enforcement agencies. The

---

[3] Johnston LD, O'Malley PM, Bachman JG & Schulenberg JE (2013). Monitoring the Future National Results on Drug Use: 2012 Overview, Key Findings on Adolescent Drug Use. Ann Arbor: Institute for Social Research, The University of Michigan.

[4] The DAWN Report, December 4, 2012.

[5] Substance Abuse and Mental Health Services Administration, Drug Abuse Warning Network, 2011: National Estimates of Drug-Related Emergency Department Visits. HHS Publication No. (SMA) 13-4760, DAWN Series D-39. Rockville, MD: Substance Abuse and Mental Health Services Administration, 2013.

abuse of these substances in the smoked form (applied to the plant material) has been corroborated by forensic laboratory analysis of products encountered by law enforcement agencies. Smoking synthetic cannabinoids for the purpose of achieving intoxication and experiencing the psychoactive effects has been identified as a reason for emergency room visits and calls to poison control centers.

Since 2009, DEA has received an increasing number of reports from poison control centers, hospitals, and law enforcement agencies concerning products containing synthetic cannabinoids. Emergency room physicians report that individuals who use these types of products experience dangerous side effects, including: convulsions, anxiety attacks, dangerously elevated heart rates, increased blood pressure, vomiting, disorientation, and hallucinations. Health warnings have been issued by numerous state and local public health departments and poison control centers describing the adverse health effects associated with the use of these synthetic cannabinoids and their related products, including agitation, anxiety, nausea, vomiting, tachycardia (fast, racing heartbeat), elevated blood pressure, tremor, seizures, hallucinations, paranoid behavior, and non-responsiveness. Because these substances pose a threat to the public health and safety, at least 45 states have taken action to control one or more of these chemicals.

From January 2010 through August 2013, poison centers in the United States have reported receiving 16,923 calls from all 50 states, Washington, DC, Puerto Rico, and overseas military or diplomatic personnel related to the exposure (closed human exposures) to synthetic marijuana (THC homologs).[6] In 2013 alone (January to August 2013), poison centers have received 1,821 calls regarding exposures (closed human exposures) to synthetic marijuana (THC homologs).[7] It is clear that they pose a significant immediate health concern that cannot be ignored.

Case reports describe acute psychotic episodes, withdrawal, and dependence associated with use of these synthetic cannabinoids, similar to syndromes observed in marijuana abuse. Based on law enforcement encounters reported directly to DEA, when responding to incidents involving individuals who have reportedly smoked these synthetic cannabinoids, first responders report that some of these individuals have suffered from intense hallucinations. Emergency department physicians and toxicologists have also reported the adverse health effects associated with smoking herbal incense products laced with these substances. Law enforcement agencies have recently reported examples of suspected *Driving Under the Influence of Drug* incidents that were attributed to the smoking of synthetic cannabinoids.

---

[6] American Association of Poison Control Centers, Synthetic Marijuana Data, August 31, 2013 (https://aapcc.s3.amazonaws.com/files/library/Synthetic_Marijuana_Data_for_Website_8.31.2013.pdf).
[7] Id.

In August 2013, eight people, ages 16 to 26, were hospitalized in Georgia due to nausea, vomiting, dry mouth, weakness, cardiac issues and paralysis after ingesting an "herbal incense" product called "Crazy Clown," a synthetic marijuana substitute that was labeled "not for human consumption." The Crazy Clown smokeable synthetic drug that caused these overdoses was sold in a retail store located in Georgia that had been raided by law enforcement earlier in the year. Following this raid, the owner was charged with distribution of a Schedule I controlled substance. On September 12, 2013, the Georgia Bureau of Investigations confirmed the presence of a new synthetic cannabinoid, ADB-PINACA, in the Crazy Clown product. This type of incident is fast becoming the norm.

In a fact sheet issued by the National Drug Court Institute, the problem of synthetic cannabinoid abuse is described as "significant and disturbing." This is supported by information that was communicated to DEA from one of the major private toxicology laboratories. Specifically, laboratory findings from drug screens for the period July 2010 through November 2010, showed over 3,700 specimens tested positive for the synthetic cannabinoids JWH-018 or JWH-073. They also indicated that they were finding 30-35% positivity for specimens submitted by juvenile probation departments.

Regulatory Control

DEA has the authority to control new designer drugs through the regulatory process, pursuant to delegated authority from the Attorney General.[8] The Comprehensive Crime Control Act of 1984 (Pub. L. 98-473), which was signed into law on October 12, 1984, amended section 201 of the CSA (21 U.S.C. § 811) to give the Attorney General the authority to temporarily place a substance into Schedule I of the CSA for one year, without regard for the requirements of 21 U.S.C. § 811(b), if he finds that such action is necessary to avoid imminent hazard to the public safety. On July 9, 2012, the President signed into law the Synthetic Drug Abuse Prevention Act of 2012 (Public Law 112-144, Title XI, Subtitle D) (SDAPA). The law placed cannabimimetic agents (any substance that is a cannabinoid receptor type I (CB-I) agonist) and 26 synthetic drugs into schedule I (15 cannabinoids, two cathinones, and nine phenethylamines); and extended the maximum time that DEA may temporarily control a substance from 12 to 24 months and increased the extension period from six months to 12 months during pendency of proceedings under 21 U.S.C. § 811(a)(1). DEA appreciates the support and hard work of this Caucus for taking the lead with this legislation to help law enforcement combat the proliferation of designer drugs. The extent and magnitude of the trafficking, regional distribution, and use of these drugs remains a problem since the passage of SDAPA and, in fact, designer drugs continue to proliferate throughout the country. SDAPA was a great starting point.

---

[8] 28 CFR § 0.100.

A substance may be temporarily scheduled under the emergency provisions of the CSA if it is not listed in any other schedule under section 202 of the CSA (21 U.S.C. § 812), and if there is no exemption or approval in effect under 21 U.S.C. § 355 for the substance.[9] DEA has utilized this authority to temporarily schedule designer drugs, but the volume of new substances that are appearing on the retail market is exploding, and DEA is constantly behind the clandestine chemists and traffickers who quickly and easily replace newly controlled substances with new, non-controlled substances. The time and resources required to collect, analyze, and study abuse data, and collect scientific evidence necessary to support a temporary scheduling action is resource intensive. While DEA supports weighing the benefits and costs of various scheduling processes and scheduling actions, we are concerned that clandestine chemists are taking advantage of the time lag. During that time period, several new drugs can appear in the marketplace replacing the drugs under review.

DEA utilized its temporary scheduling authority in March 2011to temporarily place the following five synthetic cannabinoids into Schedule I of the CSA. (76 Fed. Reg. 11075):

1-pentyl-3-(1-naphthoyl)indole (JWH-018);
1-butyl-3-(1-naphthoyl) indole (JWH-073);
1-[2-(4-morpholinyl)ethyl]-3-(1-naphthoyl)indole (JWH-200);
5-(1,1-dimethylheptyl)-2-[(1R,3S)-3-hydroxycyclohexyl]-phenol (CP-47,497); and
5-(1,1-dimethyloctyl)-2-[(1R,3S)-3-hydroxycyclohexyl]-phenol
(cannabicyclohexanol; CP- 47,497 C8 homologue).

The regulatory action to permanently schedule these substances was not completed before Congress intervened and controlled cannabimimetic agents, and these five as well as ten additional synthetic cannabinoids (AM-2201, AM-694, JWH-081, JWH-019, JWH-250, JWH-122, JWH-203, JWH-398, SR-19, and SR-18) as Schedule I substances. As will be explained in more detail later in this statement, this Congressional action conserved government resources and weakened the ability of designer drug traffickers to substitute non-controlled designer drugs for newly controlled drugs. Designer drug traffickers evade the law by staying ahead of administrative scheduling actions, and they are able to do this because of the substantial time required to support administrative scheduling.

On May 16, 2013, DEA issued a final order to temporarily schedule three more synthetic cannabinoids pursuant to 21 U.S.C. § 811(h). The substances that were the subject of the action were:

---

[9] 21 U.S.C. § 811(h).

(1-pentyl-1H-indol-3-yl)(2,2,3,3- tetramethylcyclopropyl)methanone (UR-144);
[1-(5-fluoro-pentyl)-1H- indol-3-yl](2,2,3,3-tetramethylcyclopropyl)methanone
(5-fluoro-UR-144, XLR11); and
N-(1-adamantyl)-1-pentyl-1H-indazole-3-carboxamide (APINACA, AKB48).

This action was based on a finding by the DEA that the placement of these synthetic cannabinoids and their salts, isomers and salts of isomers into Schedule I of the CSA was necessary to avoid an imminent hazard to the public safety. As a result of this order, the full effect of the CSA and the Controlled Substances Import and Export Act (CSIEA) and their implementing regulations including criminal, civil and administrative penalties, sanctions and regulatory controls of Schedule I substances were imposed on the manufacture, distribution, possession, importation, and exportation of these synthetic cannabinoids. It was approximately 15 months from the time these substances were encountered to the time the substances were temporarily controlled.

Currently, 18 synthetic cannabinoids have been controlled either through legislation or regulatory action. Unfortunately DEA has identified over 75 additional synthetic cannabinoids that are not controlled but are currently appearing in the domestic marketplace, encountered by foreign agencies, or discussed on the Internet. The ease with which foreign chemists can develop and manufacture designer drugs in clandestine laboratories located outside of the United States, creates challenges for the administrative scheduling option when dealing with large-scale manufacturing and distribution of designer drugs. As you know, Congress maintains the option to schedule designer drugs through legislation, which in the past was a quick and effective method of getting known, dangerous, synthetic substances out of the marketplace.

Synthetic Stimulants: Phenethylamines and Cathinone-type Substances

Background and History

The abuse of synthetic compounds of the phenethylamine class has also increased within the last four years. On February 1, 2011, Office of National Drug Control Policy Director Gil Kerlikowske issued a press release concerning the emerging threat of synthetic stimulants. In his statement, Director Kerlikowske stated, "I am deeply concerned about the distribution, sale and use of synthetic stimulants-especially those that are marketed as legal substances. Although we lack sufficient data to understand exactly how prevalent the use of these stimulants is, we know they pose a serious threat to the health and well-being of young people and anyone who may use them."

This class of drugs produces stimulant effects when ingested and is sometimes referred to as cathinone-type substances. The addition of a beta-keto (β-keto) substituent to the phenethylamine core structure along with substitutions on the alpha (α) carbon atom or the

11

nitrogen atom produce a group of substances called cathinones or synthetic cathinones. Cathinone is an active ingredient in the leaves of the khat plant. A number of synthetic cathinones are central nervous system stimulants.

These drugs have been trafficked and abused in Europe, particularly Great Britain and Germany, for several years. Mephedrone was first detected as a drug of abuse in Europe in November 2007. Some examples of synthetic cathinones encountered by U.S. law enforcement authorities include methcathinone, 4-methyl-N-methylcathinone (mephedrone), 3,4-methylenedioxy-N-methylcathinone (methylone), 3,4-methylenedioxypyrovalerone (MDPV), 4-methyl-N-ethylcathinone (4-MEC), 4-methyl-pyrrolidinopropiophenone (4-MePPP), alpha-pyrrolidinopentiophenone (α-PVP), beta-keto-methylbenzodioxolypentanamine (pentylone), 4-fluoro-N-methylcathinone (4-FMC), 3-fluoro-N-methylcathinone (3-FMC), napthylpyrovalerone (naphyrone), and other cathinones.

Synthetic stimulant substances are suspected to be manufactured in bulk quantities in Asian countries, and some of the actual products may be packaged for wholesale distribution in intermediate locations such as Eastern Europe. U.S. retailers sell prepackaged material or purchase it in bulk and package it under their own brand label. Products are sold at retail in a powder or crystalized form that can be easily ingested. Users self-administer the drugs by snorting the powder, smoking it, or injecting intravenously.

Similar to the synthetic cannabinoids, these substances were initially marketed as "legal" alternatives to controlled substances such as cocaine, amphetamine, ecstasy (MDMA or 3,4-methylenedioxymethamphetamine) and methcathinone. However, the marketing strategy evolved to evade criminal prosecution. Similar to the cannabinoid products, these substances are marketed as "research chemicals," "plant food," or "bath salts," and labeled "not for human consumption," in order to circumvent application of the CSA. Marketing in this manner attempts to hide the true reason for the products' existence -- the distribution of a psychoactive/stimulant substance for abuse. As with the synthetic cannabinoids, the synthetic stimulants are sold at smoke shops, head shops, convenience stores, adult book stores, gas stations, and on Internet sites. Retailers that sell these products post a disclaimer on their websites that their products are "not intended for human consumption," again, in an attempt to circumvent statutory and regulatory controls. Websites have listed products containing these synthetic stimulants as "plant food" or "bath salts," however, the powdered form is also encapsulated in gelatin capsules, and dealers offer "discreet delivery" to the potential customer. Similar to synthetic cannabinoids, law enforcement personnel have encountered dosage form and packaging operations in places such as residential neighborhoods, garages, and warehouses. There is no uniformity of drug, strength or ingredients in products of a specific brand. In fact, it is not uncommon for law enforcement personnel to seize the same brand name designer drug product in different states and find that the products contain different synthetic substances. For example, the designer drug product labeled "eight ballz glass cleaner" encountered in New Hampshire and New York in April, 2013, contained very different substances. There was no information on the product packaging, but laboratory analysis determined that the New Hampshire product contained 4-MePPP, α-PVP, benzocaine, lidocaine, and caffeine; and the New York product contained pentylone, pentedrone, α-PBP, fluoromethamphetamine, caffeine, and benzocaine. The manufacturers and distributors of these substances clearly have no concern for the adverse health consequences that may occur from ingesting the drug or combination of drugs.

Today, the list of products containing the designer stimulants has expanded to include "shoe deodorizer," "glass cleaner," and "jewelry cleaner," under brand names such as "Ivory Wave," "Purple Wave," "Vanilla Sky," "White Rush," White Girl," "White China," "Dynamite," "Bliss," "Energy-1" (NRG-1), "Ocean Snow," "Hurricane Charlie," "White Lightening," "Red Dove," "Cloud-9," "White Dove," and many others. However, the sundry items containing these drugs had nothing to do with the advertised purpose of the product. This is apparent when comparing the designer drug "bath salts," sold at retail in packages of 250mg, 500mg and 1gram, for $20 to $50, with 567 grams of genuine bath salts that can be purchased for $6-8.

Initially, three compounds, MDPV (3, 4-methylenedioxypyrovalerone), mephedrone (4-methylmethcathinone), and methylone (3,4-methylenedioxymethcathinone) were most frequently found in the U.S. marketplace. Even though DEA temporarily controlled these substances on October 21, 2011, methylone was identified in at least 145 shipments encountered by U.S. Customs and Border Protection from June 2008 to December 2012 at select U.S. ports of entry. These shipments of methylone were in powdered form, ranging from gram to multi-kilogram quantities. Most of the methylone shipments originated in China and were destined for delivery throughout the U.S. to states including Alaska, Arizona, Arkansas, California, Colorado, Florida, Hawaii, Illinois, Indiana, Kansas, Louisiana, Oklahoma, Oregon, Missouri, Nevada, New Mexico, Tennessee, Texas, Washington, and West Virginia.

Although methylone and MDPV remain in the illicit marketplace, recent intelligence and direct evidence suggest a shift to new drugs within this class that are either currently non-controlled or may be considered analogues of controlled substances including 4-MEC, 4-EMC, buphedrone, butylone, ethylone and flephedrone.

Some synthetic stimulants are known on the street by nicknames such as "Meow Meow," "drone," or "Molly." There have been several recent reports of overdose deaths associated with "Molly." The origin of the term Molly dates back several years and historically was a term used to describe the pure powder form of MDMA (3,4,methylenedioxymethamphetamine) used to manufacture (i.e., press) ecstasy pills. Prior to the MDMA being adulterated, the pure, high quality powder was often referred to as "Molly."

In the past several years, the term "Molly" has evolved to include a variety of powdered chemicals and analogues of MDMA. Law enforcement authorities have noticed the term frequently used to refer to methylone (temporarily controlled on October 21, 2011, and permanently controlled on April 12, 2013), as well as widely regarded controlled substance analogues such as 4-MEC and alpha-PVP. These designer drugs are synthesized to mimic the effects of pure MDMA and are currently being sold and distributed under the name "Molly." The DEA has seen recent multi-kilogram seizures of methylone and other widely regarded controlled substance analogues that are being sold as Molly.

On June 30, 2013, one person died and 125 were hospitalized after ingesting a drug called "Molly" while attending the Central Washington State Music Festival. At a bar in Boston, on August 28, 2013, three people overdosed, and one person died from a drug overdose from what authorities believe may have been "Molly." And on September 2, 2013, two people died and four more were hospitalized in New York City at a concert after apparently taking a drug marketed as "Molly." Toxicology reports will provide a better understanding of the causes of these deaths.

Adverse Effects

These synthetic substances are abused for their desired effects, such as euphoria, alertness, and sexual arousal. However, they cause effects similar to those of other stimulants such as methamphetamine, MDMA, and cocaine. Adverse or toxic effects associated with the abuse of phenethylamines, including synthetic cathinones, include sympathomimetic stimulation (tachycardia, hypertension, hyperthermia, mydriasis, rhabdomyolysis, hyponatremia, serotonin toxicity, and seizures), bruxism, sweating, headache, palpitations, and altered mental status (paranoia, hallucinations, delusions), and even death. Other effects that have been reported from the use of these drugs include psychological effects such as confusion, acute psychosis, combativeness, and agitation. Finally, reports of death from individuals abusing drugs in this class indicate the seriousness of the risk users are taking when ingesting these products.

In 2010, NFLIS received over 700 reports from analyzed seizures related to these substances. In 2011, it received 6,925 such reports. In 2012, NFLIS received over 14,000 reports from analyzed seizures related to 31 different synthetic cathinones. From October 2010 to June 2013, poison centers in the United States have received 9,626 calls from all 50 states, the District of Columbia, and overseas military or diplomatic personnel, related to the side effects of and overdoses from exposure to synthetic cathinone products. In 2013 alone (January to June 2013), poison centers have received 520 calls regarding exposure to synthetic cathinones.

There is very limited information regarding the biological effects of these substances, and it is unknown what may be the potential acute and long-term effects on humans. What is known about these drugs is disconcerting. There have been reports in the media of overdoses from ingestion of "bath salt" products which resulted in emergency room visits, hospitalizations, and severe psychotic episodes, some of which have led to violent outbursts, self-inflicted wounds, and, in at least one instance, suicide. Abusers of "bath salt" products have reported that they experienced many adverse effects such as chest pain, increased blood pressure, increased heart rate, agitation, panic attacks, hallucinations, extreme paranoia, and delusions. Some users have reported anecdotally that they have "crashed" or "comedown" from mephedrone with effects similar to those they experienced from "coming down" from ecstasy and cocaine.

Regulatory Control

On September 8, 2011, DEA published a Notice of Intent to temporarily place 3,4-methylenedioxy-N-methylcathinone (methylone) along with two other synthetic cathinones (4-methyl-N-methylcathinone (mephedrone) and 3,4-methylenedioxypyrovalerone (MDPV)) into Schedule I of the CSA. (76 Fed. Reg. 55616). On October 21, 2011, DEA published a Final Order temporarily placing these three synthetic cathinones into Schedule I of the CSA pursuant to the temporary scheduling provisions of 21 U.S.C. § 811(h). (76 Fed. Reg. 65371). This Final Order was based on findings by the DEA that the temporary scheduling of these three synthetic cathinones was necessary to avoid an imminent hazard to the public safety. On April 12, 2013, DEA issued a final rule placing the substance 3,4- methylenedioxy-N-methylcathinone (methylone) including its salts, isomers, and salts of isomers whenever the existence of such salts, isomers, and salts of isomers is possible, into Schedule I of the CSA.[10]

Concerns over the abuse of methylone and other synthetic cathinones have prompted many states to control these substances. As of August 2013, at least 45 states and Puerto Rico have, by legislation, banned substituted cathinones as a response to the retail sale of synthetic stimulant substances masquerading as bath salts, plant food, and glass cleaner. The Boards of Pharmacy in Oregon and Washington have added synthetic cannabinoids and substituted cathinones to their Schedule I controlled list. Additionally, the trend in the development, distribution, and consumption of this class of substances in Europe has resulted in the United Kingdom and Germany banning products containing these substances. Finally, the U.S. Armed Forces prohibits the use of synthetic cathinones including mephedrone, methylone, and MDPV.

Other Designer Drugs

Below is a brief synopsis of substances recently encountered on the designer drug market. The list is intended to provide a few examples and is not exhaustive. As mentioned earlier, the

---

[10] Mephedrone and MDPV were among the group of synthetic drugs placed in Schedule I by SDAPA on July 9, 2012. Because methylone was not included among this group, DEA continued its administrative scheduling process to permanently place methylone in Schedule I.

international community generally refers to these synthetic substances as new psychoactive substances (NPS). Among the NPS that have emerged in recent years are a range of phenethylamine analogues designed to mimic the psychostimulant properties of amphetamine, ecstasy (3,4-methylenedioxymethamphetamine, ''MDMA''), cocaine, LSD, and THC. These include amphetamine-like substances, cathinone derivatives (e.g., mephedrone), 2C compounds, piperazines, tryptamines, arylcyclohexamines (PCP-like substances and many others that include such classes as, aminoindanes, aminotetralins and benzofurans (e.g., 1-(benzofuran-5- yl) propan-2-amine (5-APB) and1-(benzofuran-6-yl)propan-2-amine hydrochloride (6-APB)— ''benzo-fury'').

<u>Phenethylamines</u>

Phenethylamines are a large class of substances that are formed by a three unit chain (ethylamine) consisting of an alpha (α) carbon atom, a beta (β) carbon atom which has a six-membered ring of carbon atoms (called a phenyl ring) attached, and a nitrogen atom that terminates the chain. The phenethylamine core chemical structure may be substituted on the nitrogen atom, at the alpha and beta carbons of the ethylamine chain, and on the phenyl ring to give rise to a myriad of substances in this chemical class. These substances affect monoaminergic transmission in the central nervous system by blocking monoaminergic uptake, releasing monoaminergic substances, or activating the monoamine receptors. These actions are believed to be involved in the stimulant and hallucinogenic effects of the phenethylamine class of drugs. Historically, a number of substances from this class of compounds have been abused for their psychoactive properties. Drugs from this class of compounds are known to produce central nervous system stimulation, visual or auditory hallucinations, or a combination of these effects. Some effects reported by abusers of phenethylamine substances include euphoria, hallucinations, sense of well-being, increased sociability, energy, empathy, increased alertness, and improved concentration and focus.

Amphetamine-like substances

Amphetamines are a class of compounds widely abused for their stimulant, euphoric, anorectic, and in some instances, emphathogenic, entactogenic, and hallucinogenic properties. These compounds derive from the b-phenethylamine core structure, they are widely characterized as synthetic drugs, of which amphetamine, methamphetamine, and 3,4-methylenedioxyamphetamine (MDMA) are some of the most well-known. The amphetamine structure allows for a number of substitutions at the aromatic ring, at the α and β positions on the aliphatic chain and the amine to give a wide range of amphetamines.

Adverse health effects continue to be a cause for emergency department presentations. Some of the substances encountered on the designer drug market include 4-fluoro-amphetamine, 4-fluoro-methamphetamine, N-ethylamphetamine, 4-methylthio-amphetamine (4-MTA), para-methoxy-methamphetamine (PMMA), and others.

2C Series Compounds

The phenethylamine core chemical structure may also be substituted on the phenyl ring at the 2-, 4- and 5-positions or the alpha (α) carbon to produce a group of substances called phenalkylamine hallucinogens. The 2- and 5-positions are typically substituted with a methoxy (-OCH3) group; whereas, the 4-position is substituted with various moieties like halogen or alkyl groups. Most of the currently known compounds of the 2C family were first synthesized by Alexander Shulgin in the 1970s and 1980s and published in his book <u>PiHKAL</u> <u>("Phenethylamines i Have Known And Loved")</u>. A number of substances from this class of compounds have been abused for their psychoactive properties.

Serotonin (5-HT)2A receptor is thought to be the primary site mediating the hallucinogenic effects of LSD and phenalkylamine hallucinogens. Some adverse health effects reported by abusers of these substances include tachycardia, hypertension, agitation, aggression, visual and auditory hallucinations, seizures, hyperpyrexia, clonus, elevated white cell count, elevated creatine kinase, metabolic acidosis, rhabdomyolysis, acute kidney injury, visual, auditory and thought process alterations, euphoria, relaxation, anxiety, paranoia, fear and dyspnea (breathing difficulty), nausea, vomiting, and mydriasis (dilation of pupils). There have been reports of emergency room admissions and deaths associated with abuse of phenethylamine substances.

Some examples of these substances encountered include 2,5-dimethoxy-4-iodophenethylamine (2C-I), 2,5-dimethoxy-4-ethylthiophenethylamine (2C-T-2) and 1-(2,5-dimethoxy-4-iodophenyl)-2-aminopropane (DOI) 2,5-dimethoxy-4-bromophenethylamine (2C-B), 2,5-dimethoxy-4-propylthiophenethylamine (2C-T-7), 2-(4-Iodo-2,5-dimethoxyphenyl)-N-(2-methoxybenzyl)ethanamine (25I-NBOMe), 2,5-dimethoxy-4-bromoamphetamine (DOB), and 2,5-dimethoxy–4-methylamphetamine (DOM). These substances are primarily abused for their hallucinogenic-like effects and are often promoted as legal alternatives to ecstasy or lysergic acid diethylamide (LSD).

Under SDAPA, nine 2C compounds were placed in Schedule I and at approximately the same time, a rapid increase in encounters of other 2C compounds was experienced. Of these, 25I-NBOMe, 25C-NBOMe, and 25B-NBOMe were encountered in powder form, on blotter paper and in eye-dropper bottles, to name a few, and the abuse of these substances has been connected to a number of serious adverse health effects. With no approved medical use, these synthetic phenethylamines are mainly abused for their hallucinogenic effects and are purported to be active at extremely low dosages, especially the NBOMe-functionalized 2C series, and have been found to produce severe clinical toxicities.

Abuse of 25I-NBOMe, 25C-NBOMe and 25B-NBOMe has been characterized with acute public health and safety issues both domestically and abroad (Advisory Council on the Misuse of Drugs, 2013). NFLIS has a total of 689 drug reports (June 2011 through March 2013) in which 25I-NBOMe, 25C-NBOMe or 25B-NBOMe were identified from a number of states including, Alabama, Arkansas, California, Colorado, Connecticut, Florida, Georgia, Iowa, Indiana, Illinois, Kansas, Kentucky, Louisiana, Maryland, Maine, Minnesota, Missouri, New Hampshire, New Jersey, New Mexico, North Dakota, Nebraska, Nevada, Ohio, Oklahoma,

Pennsylvania, South Carolina, Tennessee, Texas, Utah, Virginia, Wisconsin and Wyoming as of March 2013. (query date: August 7, 2013). As of August 16, 2013, a number of states, including Arkansas, Florida, Louisiana, Nebraska, Ohio, Utah and Virginia have controlled one or more of these substances. Abuse of these substances abroad has prompted the United Kingdom, Israel, and Russia to control these substances as well.

25I-NBOMe was developed as a research chemical in 2003, but had nearly no history of human use before 2010, when it first became available online. It is sometimes compared to LSD because it is a hallucinogen and it is often sold on blotter paper or in dropper bottles, rather than sold as a pill or in powder form. 25I-NBOMe is not generally sold in commercial retail environments, but is readily available on the Internet and is often mailed in distribution quantities to the buyer for subsequent resale. Then it is often sold individually for approximately $5-$10 per dosage unit (on blotter paper or in dropper bottles). It is much stronger than most of the 2C-phenethylamines – dosage units are in micrograms rather than milligrams. This potency level makes it extremely hazardous to unsuspecting users. Lack of knowledge about this drug was likely at least partially responsible for 14 deaths that occurred in a 14-month time span 2012 and 2013. These documented deaths occurred in California, Texas, Tennessee, Louisiana, North Dakota, North Carolina, Alabama, West Virginia, Florida and Ohio. Unconfirmed Medical Examiner/Toxicology reports list another 13 deaths in the United States that may be attributed to 25I-NBOMe.

Piperazines

Piperazines are a class of compounds that share a core benzylpiperazine chemical structure. N-Benzylpiperazine (BZP) and 1-(3-trifluoromethylphenyl)piperazine (TFMPP) are the two most commonly encountered by law enforcement. BZP and TFMPP are promoted mainly in combination as legal alternatives to 3,4-methylenedioxy-methamphetamine (MDMA) and are often sold as "Ecstasy," "legal E" or "legal X". The piperazines can produce a wide range of effects including central nervous system stimulation or hallucinations. Like amphetamine and MDMA, the effects of BZP are stimulant-like while those of TFMPP are hallucinogen like. BZP acts as a stimulant similar in effects to a low dose of MDMA or amphetamine, producing euphoria and inducing cardiovascular effects, including increased heart rate, systolic blood pressure and pulse rate. TFMPP is a serotonin releasing agent and binds to serotonin receptors in the brain.

Tryptamines

Tryptamines are a class of substances that consists of an indole ring connected to a two carbon (ethyl) chain with a terminal nitrogen atom. Tryptamines have an indole ring structure joined to an amino group by a 2 carbon side chain. Substitutions at various positions on the indole ring and the alpha (α) and beta (β) carbons with carbon-containing moieties give rise to various tryptamine compounds. Serotonin (5-HT) 2A receptor is thought to be the primary site mediating the hallucinogenic effects these substances. Some tryptamines encountered by law enforcement include 5-methoxy-N,N-diallyltryptamine (5-MeO-DALT), 5-methoxy-N,N-dimethyltryptamine (5-MeO-DMT), 5-methoxy-N,N-diethyltryptamine (5-MeO-DET), 5-methoxy-N,N-alphamethyltryptamine (5-MeO-AMT), N,N-diisopropyltryptamine (DIPT), 4-

hydroxy-N,N-diisopropyltryptamine (4-OH-DIPT), 4-hydroxy-N-methyl-N-isopropyltryptamine (4-OH-MiPT; miprocin),5-methoxy-N-methyl-N-isopropyltryptamine (5-MeO-MIPT), alpha-ethyltryptamine (AET), N,N-dimethyltryptamine (DMT), N,N-diethyltryptamine (DET), bufotenine, psilocybin,psilocin, and others.

These substances are abused for their hallucinogenic-like effects and can produce adverse health effects. Some adverse effects reported include experiencing restlessness, mental activation, nervousness, changes in auditory, visual, and gustatory perceptions, intense emotions, insight, distorted reality, alteration of sensory perception and judgment, and fear. These can pose serious health risks to the user and the general public. There have been reports of emergency room admissions and deaths associated with the abuse of these substances.

Arylcyclohexamines

Arylcyclohexamines encompass a group of synthetic psychoactive substances which are structurally and pharmacologically similar to ketamine, phencyclidine (PCP), and N-ethyl-1-phenylcyclohexylamine (PCE), a Schedule I drug. PCP effects are unpredictable. PCP is known for its ability to produce violent behavior. High doses of PCP are known to produce convulsions, coma, hyperthermia and death. Ketamine and phencyclidine are "club drugs" and they produce feelings of detachment or dissociation from the environment or self in users. The arylcycloheaxmines that are currently being abused are methoxetamine (MXE), 3-methoxy-PCE, 3-methoxy-PCP, and 4-methoxy-PCP. Pharmacological studies have shown that these four substances act comparably to PCP and ketamine at the cellular level.

Of these four substances, MXE is being abused at the highest rate. MXE is generally abused for its hallucinogenic and dissociative effects. Users administer the drug by snorting, applying under the tongue, injecting intravenously or intramuscularly. Users report experiencing mild euphoria, hallucinations, disorientation, confusion and anxiety. In a drug discrimination study MXE mimicked PCP in its effects in rats that were trained to recognize PCP from saline. In this study, MXE was about 2.5-fold more potent than PCP.[11] There have been reports of overdoses from MXE toxicity and one confirmed death in the U.S. has been reported in which MXE was determined to be the cause of death. Multiple deaths have been attributed to MXE in Europe.

Current Efforts and Challenges

Current efforts to stem the rising distribution and abuse of hundreds of designer drugs include controlling each substance through the administrative rulemaking process (temporarily and/or permanently) and prosecuting individual violators pursuant to the Analogue Act. Each

---

[11] Fantegrossi, WE, Novel eticyclidine analogues as emerging drugs of abuse, 75th Annual Meeting - College on Problems of Drug Dependence - June 14-19, 2013, San Diego, CA.

approach presents resource challenges to efforts to protect the public from these dangerous substances.

Scheduling by Administrative Rulemaking: Temporary Control

By their nature, designer drugs are non-controlled substances. They can be controlled under the CSA either by Congress or by DEA through its administrative rulemaking authority. DEA may also temporarily place a substance into Schedule I of the CSA for a maximum of three years if such action is necessary to avoid imminent hazard to the public safety, it is not listed in any other schedule under section 202 of the CSA (21 U.S.C. § 812), and if there is no exemption or approval in effect under 21 U.S.C. § 355 for the substance. As described above, DEA has utilized its regulatory authority to place many synthetic cannabinoids and synthetic stimulants into the CSA pursuant to its temporary scheduling authority. Once a substance is temporarily controlled, DEA moves towards permanent control by requesting a scientific and medical evaluation from the Department of Health and Human Services, and gathering and analyzing additional scientific data and other information collected from all sources, including poison control centers, hospitals, and law enforcement agencies, in order to consider the additional factors warranting its permanent control.

DEA is constantly gathering scientific data and other relevant information about other designer drugs as well as evaluating their psychoactive effects to support administrative action to control these substances under the CSA. The time and resources required to collect, analyze, and study abuse data, and collect scientific evidence necessary to support temporary and permanent scheduling actions is substantial, and, in recent years, addressing designer drugs has resulted in DEA re-prioritizing its resources.

In 2010 and 2011, these substances were an emerging public safety threat requiring the DEA to devote a large amount of its resources to compiling the necessary scientific data and information, initiate control actions and communicate the scientific and technical information with other offices within DEA and other Federal agencies. The DEA staff in the Office of Diversion Control are responsible for drug scheduling actions also coordinates the rulemaking process to designate anabolic steroids that are subject to control under the CSA. It is responsible for conducting studies and evaluations pertaining to all aspects of drug control and chemical regulation. It initiates studies to increase and apply scientific knowledge concerning the scheduling and rescheduling of controlled substances and the regulation of chemicals and precursors. This section monitors and documents abuse and law enforcement encounters with illicit and emerging drugs of abuse. It collaborates with other agencies within the U.S. government and outside of the government (e.g., academic institutions) to obtain necessary scientific information to evaluate drugs for possible control under the CSA. It conducts pharmacological reviews on drugs that are the subject of either a request for control status determination under the CSA or for a controlled substance analogue determination. It serves as a point of contact for the DEA and outside organizations for technical and regulatory control information on drugs of abuse. This section manages information and data collection programs including NFLIS. It analyzes and interprets information and data from various data sources, and prepares reports of drug abuse and chemical diversion emergent and changing trends.

Due to the designer drug problem, DEA's administrative scheduling actions have increased and the responsibilities of the scientific staff have expanded. There is expanding need for educational efforts across the country. In 2010, DEA scientific staff provided four presentations on designer drugs; in 2011, they presented seven times; in 2012, they presented 11 times; and as of August 21, 2013, they have already given ten presentations. These presentations were provided to various scientific and professional organizations, both domestic and abroad, domestic law enforcement personnel and organizations, as well as the international control community.

This developed expertise has demanded scientific staff testimony in important criminal prosecutions of traffickers of these dangerous synthetic drugs. This is a relatively recent, growing responsibility and is stretching the resources of the scientific staff as they conduct the scientific analysis required as well as provide expert testimony in numerous criminal prosecutions brought under the Analogue Act.

From 1997 to 2010, DEA temporarily scheduled a total of four substances in 2002 and 2003, in order to avoid imminent hazard to the public safety pursuant to 21 U.S.C. § 811(h). As discussed, in 2011, DEA began to use its temporary scheduling authority to control numerous emerging designer drugs because there was a marked increase in the trafficking and abuse of illicit designer drugs such as synthetic cannabinoids and cathinones. In 2011, DEA temporarily scheduled eight synthetic substances and subsequently prepared to permanently control these substances. In 2012, DEA was working towards permanently controlling the eight temporarily controlled designer drugs from 2011, and published NPRMs for six of those substances. Also in 2012, scientific staff provided expert testimony in ten instances and provided technical support in 18 instances with respect to Analogue Act prosecutions. By the end of August 2013, DEA had temporarily controlled three more synthetic designer drugs, while the scientific staff has provided testimony in 32 instances, and were providing technical support (including written declarations) in approximately 135 instances, all in support of Analogue Act criminal prosecutions.

Since FY 2012, the DEA laboratory system has experienced a growth in the proportion of synthetic cannabinoid and synthetic cathinone drug exhibits submitted to the laboratories. In FY 2011, synthetic compounds accounted for less than 1 percent of total drug submissions to DEA labs for forensic analysis. By FY 2012, this figure grew to 22 percent of submitted drug exhibits and is on pace to account for over 14 percent of drug exhibits submitted to the laboratory in FY 2013. Submissions of synthetic compounds largely contributed to an overall increase of approximately 15,000 exhibits to the DEA laboratory system in FY 2012, pushing backlog levels over 20,000 exhibits, well over the historically manageable 10,000-exhibit level.

Based upon current staffing levels and barring unforeseen circumstances, DEA's seven field laboratories are capable of analyzing approximately 54,000 exhibits annually. In FY 2012, the DEA field laboratories received over 68,000 exhibits, and they are projected to receive approximately the same amount of exhibits in FY 2013. At this rate and barring any mitigation strategies, system's backlog could reach 30,000 exhibits by the end of CY 2013.

In addition to the strain on laboratories and scientific staff, the current approach to the designer drug problem comes at a high cost to the government. For example, a recent purchase of a group of reference standards for analytical testing was approximately $300,000. And, DEA spent approximately $335,000 in hazardous and toxic waste clean-up costs related to Operation Log Jam and Operation Synergy (discussed below).

The abuse of designer drugs also results in additional costs for companies conducting routine drug screens, hospitals, and others attempting to monitor and connect an adverse health event to a specific substance. Generally, time is required to develop methods for detection in response to designer drug abuse.

The greatest concern is the toll designer drug trafficking takes on our citizens and our communities, and the burden on the healthcare system. For example, an emergency room physician recently stated that of 179 patients admitted to the Intensive Care Unit after ingesting designer drugs, only four had health insurance. Furthermore, his emergency room was forced to employ a full-time, armed security guard to protect the medical personnel from these patients who are routinely combative and/or suffer from acute psychotic episodes.[12]

During the time period DEA is gathering information to support administrative scheduling actions, several new drugs can appear in the marketplace replacing the drugs under review. In every drug class described above, there are a number of replacement substances that could easily be substituted into over-the-counter products or as legal substitutes to controlled drugs. In fact, currently there may be in excess of 200 compounds that are suspected synthetic cannabinoids, synthetic stimulants, or synthetic hallucinogens. Although DEA utilizes its authority to temporarily schedule designer drugs, the volume of new substances that are appearing on the retail market is exploding, and DEA is constantly behind the clandestine chemists and traffickers who quickly and easily replace newly controlled substances with new,

---

[12] Presentation of Sullivan K. Smith, M.D., DEA-sponsored conference entitled "The Dangers of Designer Synthetic Drugs," August 8, 2013.

non-controlled substances. Accordingly, the administrative scheduling process by itself is not the answer to address the widespread distribution of designer drugs.

Prosecutions Pursuant to the Analogue Act

A designer drug may or may not be a "controlled substance analogue" pursuant to the CSA. Even if a particular substance is widely regarded as a "controlled substance analogue" under the CSA, each criminal prosecution must establish that fact anew. The primary challenge to preventing the distribution and abuse of a controlled substance analogue, as opposed to a controlled substance *per se*, is that the latter is specifically identified (by statute or regulation) as a controlled substance to which clear statutory controls automatically attach, while the former is not specifically identified (by statute or regulation) and is not automatically subject to control. In Analogue Act prosecutions, the government must establish that the substance involved is a "controlled substance analogue" as defined by the CSA; accordingly, each prosecution is a new case even if the same substance is involved.

The above considerations, along with the increasing volume and endless variety of designer drugs available today and the sophisticated methods and routes of distribution, render the Controlled Substance Analogue Enforcement Act ineffective by itself as a tool to prevent diversion and abuse of designer drugs. In the past, SDAPA's control of specific, known, synthetic substances was a swift and aggressive contribution to the overall effort to combat the designer drug threat.

Enforcement Operations

Even though there is no evidence of legitimate non-research related uses for these designer drugs, multiple shipments of JWH-018 and JWH-073 were encountered by U.S. Customs and Border Protection (CBP) in 2010. One enforcement operation encountered five shipments of JWH-018 totaling over 50 kilograms (110.2 pounds) of powder. In addition, bulk quantities of JWH-018 and JWH-200 were encountered by law enforcement in 2010. The CBP continues to make significant seizures of synthetic designer drugs. At just one laboratory, from May 18, 2013, until August 22, 2013, the CBP encountered over 50 kilograms of synthetic cannabinoid powder, which consisted of XLR-11, AM2201, PB-22, and 5-fluoro-PB22 in 38 shipments. And, over 21 kilograms of synthetic cathinones; including methylone, 4-MEC, alpha-PVT and alpha-PVP were encountered in 42 shipments.

DEA's Operation Log Jam was initiated in 2011 and culminated in a nationwide takedown on July 25, 2012. This operation was coordinated by DEA in cooperation with U.S. Immigration and Customs Enforcement's Homeland Security Investigations (HSI), Federal Bureau of Investigations (FBI), CBP, and the Internal Revenue Service (IRS). The goals of this operation included the targeting of manufacturers, wholesale distributors and retail distributors of designer drug products, the development of information on foreign based sources of supply, raising public awareness of the dangers associated with the use of these drugs and the development of leads for a Phase II initiative (Operation Synergy).

Operation Log Jam resulted in 100 arrests; the execution of 300 search warrants and 80 consent searches at; and the identification of 38 manufacturing sites. Law enforcement seized 196 kilograms of raw synthetic cathinones, 722 kilograms of raw synthetic cannabinoids, 167,187 packets of synthetic cathinones ready for distribution, 4,852,099 packets of synthetic cannabinoids ready for distribution, 4,766 kilograms of plant material treated with synthetic cannabinoids ready to be packaged, 21,933 kilograms of untreated plant material, over $45,000,000 in U.S. Currency and bank accounts, 88 vehicles, 77 firearms, additional assets valued at $5,688,500 and 1,096 gallons of acetone.

The information and evidence obtained during Operation Log Jam led investigators to initiate Project Synergy, the second phase of a national cooperative effort in combating the synthetic designer drug distribution. Project Synergy began in December 2012 and culminated in a nationwide take down on June 26, 2013 conducted by the DEA, HSI, FBI, CBP, and the IRS as well as domestic law enforcement departments in 45 states. This operation also included some of our international partners with joint operations being conducted with Australia, New Zealand, Canada, and Barbados.

As part of Project Synergy, the DEA conducted an enforcement operation in June 2013 in the Houston, Texas, area on a synthetic cannabinoid wholesale distributor who was selling AM-2201 and XLR11. During this operation, law enforcement seized enough synthetic cannabinoid products to gross approximately $21,000,000 in revenue at the retail level. Through the course of this investigation, the manager of this operation told undercover DEA agents that he initially invested $80,000 and turned it into $6 million. This person also told the undercover agent that he makes 130 percent profit in a week and "you can't rob banks and make this kind of money."

Project Synergy involved many investigations that culminated on June 26, 2013, and included 234 arrests, 416 search warrants and 68 consent searches that led to the seizure of 305 kilograms of raw synthetic cathinones; 1,278 kilograms of raw synthetic cannabinoids; 10,263 packets of synthetic cathinones and cannabinoids; 959 kilograms of treated plant material ready to be packaged; $53,201,595 in currency and assets, 132 vehicles and 141 weapons.

Traffickers Adapting to the Law

Even though several of these designer drug compounds have been controlled/banned in most states and temporarily scheduled by DEA, entrepreneurs procure new synthetic cannabinoid compounds, which have comparative psychoactive properties, with relative ease. Clandestine chemists can easily continue to provide retailers with "legal" products by developing/synthesizing new synthetic cannabinoid products that are not controlled. In fact, after DEA took action to temporarily schedule five synthetic cannabinoids in March 2011, retailers began selling new versions of the products that did not contain the controlled cannabinoids, but instead new versions of the compounds. Retailers were provided with spurious chemical analyses that purported to document that the new product line did not contain any of the controlled cannabinoids.

In Kansas, a major manufacturer/distributor of synthetic cannabinoid products told a law enforcement officer that ". . . if the compound that he is using [JWH-250] is banned, he would just switch and treat his dried plant material with another legal compound."[13] There may be in excess of 100 synthetic cannabinoid products that have yet to be introduced into the marketplace. Manufacturers and distributors will continue to stay one step ahead of any state or Federal drug-specific banning or control action by introducing/repackaging new cannabinoid products that are not controlled.

There are also financial incentives that drive the wholesale and retail distribution of these products. Affidavits were filed by Plaintiffs in the United States District Court, District of Minnesota, in support of a motion for preliminary injunction and restraining order that attempted to enjoin the government from proceeding with the temporary scheduling of JWH-018, JWH-073, JWH-200, CP-47,497 and cannabicyclohexanol.[14] Each of the Plaintiffs, in a sworn affidavit, claimed that "outlawing" synthetic cannabinoids would have detrimental effects on their respective businesses. In total, these four Plaintiffs estimated their gross profit from the sale of these products to be in excess of $3.5 million annually. They stated that the sale of cannabinoid products represented more than 50 percent of total sales of L.P.O.E., Inc., a Minnesota corporation; more than 70 percent of total sales of Hideaway, Inc; approximately 41.27 percent of gross profits (from April 2010 to September 2010) of Down in the Valley, Inc; and approximately 57 percent of Disc and Tape, Inc sales (affiant estimated that he would lose over $6,000 per day in sales if he had to stop selling the product).

It is clear that the income generated from distributing these products is, and will continue to be, a driving factor for manufacturers, distributors, and retailers to seek/find substitute products that are not yet controlled or banned by Federal or state action. This is reminiscent of the typical illicit drug dealer cost-benefit analysis, in which the potential for financial gain far outweighs the potential for legal consequences especially in the controlled substance analogue arena. The large profits and the fact that these chemicals can be easily synthesized to stay one

---

[13] Testimony of Police Chief James D. Hill, City of Salina, Kansas Association of Chiefs of Police Representative before the Kansas Senate Committee on Public Health and Welfare, March 3, 2011.
[14] L.P.O.E, Inc v. U.S. Drug Enforcement Administration (Civil Case No. 10-VC-4944).

step ahead of control, indicate there is no incentive to discontinue retail distribution of synthetic cannabinoid products under the current statutory and regulatory scheme. Although many good corporate citizen retailers will discontinue the sale of these products in support of public health and safety, many will not, instead opting for the profits realized to help their financial bottom line.

Outreach

Since 2010, DEA has provided awareness training, briefings and written materials to law enforcement, organizations that represent health professionals, state and Federal legislators and community groups/general public concerning new and emerging synthetic drugs. DEA representatives have briefed groups and organizations such as the International Association of Chiefs of Police, National Narcotics Officers Coalitions of America and their individual state chapters, the National Methamphetamine and Pharmaceutical Initiative, professional sports leagues, and the Community Anti-Drug Coalitions of America (CADCA) to provide information concerning the wide spectrum of synthetic drugs in the marketplace, distribution and trafficking patterns, methods of abuse and identified/reported adverse health effects. In FY 2010, DEA provided 23 presentations; in FY 2011, 30; in FY 2012, 60; and as of September 4, 2013, DEA has provided 32 presentations.

Health professionals see first-hand the carnage left in the wake of the abuse of these drugs. DEA continues to work synthetic drugs into presentations to health care professionals, and has incorporated a block of instruction into the Pharmacy Diversion Awareness Conferences given to pharmacists throughout the United States. Pharmacists are the drug experts in the healthcare delivery system, so it makes sense that they are aware of the dangers associated with these drugs.

DEA continues to use the Internet to post information concerning synthetic drugs. www.justthinktwice.com is a website for teens and young adults that provides factual information about drugs of abuse and the consequences associated with the abuse of these substances. DEA also provides information, PowerPoint presentations, videos and educational materials concerning synthetic drugs and other licit/illicit drugs of abuse for parents and educators through the DEA resource for parents, *"Get Smart About Drugs,"* that can be found as a link from the www.DEA.gov website. The DEA website also has a section dedicated to drug fact sheets for drugs of abuse including synthetic drugs.

DEA is working with our state and local partners to provide parents with the most up-to date information concerning these substances. For example, DEA has partnered with Sheriff Michael Chapman and the Loudon County Virginia Sheriff's Office to provide a series of programs for parents to learn about the abuse of synthetic designer drugs and controlled substance pharmaceuticals and allow parents the opportunity to ask questions, with the goal of formulating strategies to combat the abuse of these substances within their communities.

Finally, we acknowledge that synthetic drug products continue to be sold from gas stations and convenience stores throughout the country. In June 2013, DEA sent a letter to each of the top 100 retail convenience store and gas station chain corporations in the United States informing them of the alarming trend of the sale and abuse of synthetic designer drugs masquerading as over-the counter household items such as bath salts, incense or jewelry cleaner. The letter discussed why they are marketed and sold at retail, how they are abused and the health consequences and the dangers associated with the abuse of these substances. The letter requested that these corporations take steps to protect the public by preventing these substances from being sold at their business locations.

These corporations were then invited to attend a seminar in Arlington, Virginia on August 8, 2013 that provided a more in-depth program about the synthetic drug problem. The program, entitled, "The Dangers of Designer Synthetic Drugs" educated the participants about the dangers and consequences of selling these substances as well as to help them identify these types of products. Only four corporations attended the seminar. However, the four companies (Shell Oil, Marathon Petroleum, Citgo, and TA-Petro) have a large number of retail outlets throughout the United States and one corporation that has a network of over 14,000 branded stations in the United States indicated they were taking proactive measures in demanding that if these products are being sold in their stores, they are taken off of the shelves immediately.

Our outreach efforts to impact this threat extend to the international arena as well. In the past two years the U.S. has joined with its international partners at the yearly U.S. Commission on Narcotic Drug (CND) meetings to help formulate and advance resolutions that address the synthetic drug threat on a global level. Building on the resolution from 2012, at the March 2013 CND the U.S. was a cosponsor of a resolution entitled *"Enhancing International Cooperation in the Identification & Reporting of NPS."* Among other things, this resolution encourages nations to take a comprehensive and coordinated approach to the detection, analysis, and identification of NPS; urges nations to share with one another information on the identification of NPS using, where appropriate, existing national and regional early warning systems and networks; urges nations to include information on the potential adverse impacts and risks to public health and safety of new psychoactive substances through prevention and awareness to counter public perceptions of NPS; encourages nations, and relevant international institutions, to share and exchange ideas, best practices, and experiences regarding new laws, regulations and restrictions, to attack the NPS issue; and urges the UNODC to continue to develop a voluntary electronic portal for national forensic and/or drug testing laboratories to enable timely and comprehensive sharing of information on NPS (an early warning system).

Conclusion

The creation, manufacture and distribution of designer synthetic drugs have been an ongoing problem for decades. However, the last 5 years has brought about a new marketing and distribution strategy that has increased availability through established and defined distribution networks and overt retail sales through convenience stores, gas stations, tobacco/smoke/head shops and the Internet. This strategy has been successful as evidenced by submissions of exhibits to forensic labs, calls to poison control centers and emergency room visits. The fact that one cannabinoid, AM-2201is ranked 8th in drug submissions in NFLIS is a telling sign that these products have taken a more predominant role as drugs of abuse. The designer drug problem has grown from the small number of domestic clandestine chemists in the 1970s, 1980s and 1990s that were distributing locally/regionally to the current situation that is defined by foreign chemists and clandestine labs supplying bulk drugs to domestic wholesalers/re-packagers with sophisticated distribution chains that can get the drugs on the shelves of retail outlets in a very short period of time. Retailers are generating huge profits in the sale of these products with little concern for the safety of the public.

Clandestine chemists have created an unlimited supply of new products that will replace existing designer products when they are eventually controlled. The challenge to controlling these substances individually through administrative actions pursuant to the CSA is that the manufacturers of these substances circumvent the statutory criteria by manipulating the chemical structure of the compound. They can create substances that are pharmacologically similar to a schedule I or II controlled substance, that may or may not be chemically (structurally) similar to a schedule I or II controlled substance. The statute requires both pharmacological and chemical similarity in order to be an analogue. Even more alarming is that the structure of a chemical substance can be manipulated in endless variations while the pharmacological activity of the substance may increase or remain substantially unchanged. As a result, it is almost impossible outside of a controlled laboratory environment to determine the chemical composition, and the quantity, potency, and type of synthetic ingredients in these substances. It is equally challenging to determine what the potential harmful effects may be due to human consumption.

Our experience is that enforcement of the Analogue Act with respect to the current designer drug threat presents substantial challenges. The increasing number of designer drugs available to the public increases the time and resources necessary to administratively control these substances and to prosecute violators. Even though the individual states have legislatively controlled certain designer drugs, violators simply move their products to other states where the substances are not controlled. This caucus convened a hearing in April 2011 entitled, "The Dangers of Synthetic Cannabinoids and Stimulants." That hearing focused on several drugs in the cannabinoid (e.g., JWH compounds) and cathinone-like stimulant classes (e.g., methylone, mephedrone and MDPV) and to a lesser extent, 2C products (e.g., dimethoxyphenethylamines). Congress, under the leadership and guidance of this committee, subsequently passed the Synthetic Drug Abuse Prevention Act of 2012 (SDAPA) to address the problem. While this legislation was a great first step because it immediately controlled 26 synthetic designer drugs as Schedule I controlled substances, , today the number of identified synthetic designer drugs of all classes in the marketplace or identified but not yet encountered by law enforcement exceeds 250 compounds and includes cannabinoids, stimulants, hallucinogens, and depressants. (A list of all DEA-identified synthetic substances currently in the domestic drug market is available upon request.) Since SDAPA was enacted, our enforcement actions have increased and our prosecutions pursuant to the Analogue Act have increased because unscrupulous chemists continue to synthesize new substances faster than we can control them. The public health and safety is at risk during the time required to take action, and the injuries and deaths related to these compounds continue and are highly concerning. We appreciate the tools the Congress has given us thus far and we have made progress against certain synthetic drugs, but more work is necessary. We look forward to continuing our partnership with Congress in this area because in the past, SDAPA worked to stem the distribution and abuse of the 26 substances legislatively controlled.

In closing, the purveyors of this poison have honed their skills and learned to adapt from mistakes made in the past, and this ability to adapt has placed law enforcement and regulators at an extreme disadvantage in attempting to stop the flow of these drugs into our communities. In the meantime, our children and young adults are used as laboratory experiments by clandestine chemists and domestic profiteers looking for the next non-controlled designer drug that will be a multi-million dollar revenue generator. DEA and our state and local enforcement and regulatory partners are committed to using all of the civil, administrative, and criminal authorities at our disposal to combat the distribution of these substances, but the seemingly never ending supply of new substances is resource intensive and impacts our capacity to address other critical areas of concern.

Thank you for the opportunity to testify before the caucus today, and we look forward to working together with the Caucus as well as our local, state, tribal, and federal counterparts to protect the public against the dangers of these ever-changing synthetic designer drugs.

www.ingramcontent.com/pod-product-compliance
Lightning Source LLC
Chambersburg PA
CBHW080624180526
45168CB00007B/3049

* 9 7 8 1 5 0 8 6 0 5 7 9 9 *